Beyond Diets Program For Beginners:

Lose Weight, Burn Fat, Get a Slim Body, Increase Energy and Live Healthy

By

Valerie Alston

Table of Contents

Beyond Diet Program For Beginners: Lose Weight, Burn Fat, Get a Slim Body, Increase Energy and Live Healthy

By Valerie Alston

Introduction

Rather than focusing on the diet, Beyond Diet is a program that seeks to help the user change the lifestyle into a healthier, more fulfilling life. Rather than describing how and why one needs to go on diet, the program helps one change his or her thinking and eating habits.

The program seeks to do what many diet plans have so miserably failed to do, help everybody lose weight and live healthily. The plan therefore is like a manual that clarifies what true nutrition is and what foods should and should not be eaten so as to achieve an ideal weight and to avoid the many lifestyle diseases that are related to bad eating habits.

The plan was fashioned by a nutritionist that has had first-hand experience with many diet plans and thus understands the principles that will and will not work. She has incorporated the best principles into a single plan that is guaranteed to help in achieving optimum weight and health.

Chapter 1. Understanding The Program and Making It Work

Beyond Diet plan is for everyone especially people who have tried several diets and exercises without achieving their goals. It is a new, fresh way of living rather than a diet plan. It is easy to adjust to, and in case you have tried fitting into a diet program before, you probably know that all that is required is commitment.

Many diet programs fail because people only change what they eat without really improving their eating habits. As soon as they leave the diet program, they reverse everything the diet program helped achieve through unhealthy eating habits. Additionally, most diets rarely focus on overall health of the body. The main principle is controlled starvation. Controlled Starvation slows the body's metabolism and comes with many undesirable effects such as fatigue, increased hunger and sluggishness. Soon after you are out of a diet that works through controlled starvation, you gain weight since the metabolism of the body picks up again.

The Beyond diet aims at improving health and changing eating habits so that the effects gained are permanent. Rather than being a temporary modification of the diet, this is a permanent adjustment to your life to enhance health and achieve the ideal weight. It comes as a commitment to remain healthy and happy.

The beyond diet is not an overnight experience; it may take some time to release its full potential. However once realized, these effects will be permanent. As it is, the program is not a crash program but rather it is a lifestyle change that won't require you to give up all your favorite foods. The Beyond Diet program helps you understand where to fit your favorite foods into your program so as to enjoy them and at the same time maintain your weight and health.

The Beyond Diet is not a strict program that has to be followed verbatim for it to be effective. Those who find it hard to follow every principle should in no way feel disheartened. In any case, the program advocates for a person to take the reins of his or her health one step at a time. As long as one can stick to the principles of the program in short-term they will with time become permanent life principles which greatly benefit health.

The program begins with making a choice about where you would like to be in terms of health and weight.

Making the program work

Enjoying the success of this program will take much more than merely following the nutritional guidelines. Remember it is more than a diet plan it is a lifestyle adjustment that is meant to have a long-lasting impact on your vigor and life, in general. It is thus important to first create a positive foundation upon which you the achievement of your goals will be set.

Preconditioning the mind

The media is full of misleading info and hype that may impede the success of the program. It is thus important that you first wash your mind clean of all the hype that media may have fed you regarding diet programs. This implies that you ought not take everything a certain nutritionist or doctor says on a TV show to be the gospel truth. Disregard everything else that you have acquired from other diet plans. This, as we mentioned, is not a diet plan; it is a lifestyle adjustment. It is not only meant to help in weight management but is focused on improving your overall health.

Besides, if previous diets programs have lead you to the same unhappiness and unhealthy weight conditions, why should you pay attention to them?

Have faith

Beyond Diet can only be optimally successful if one has faith in the program as well as a firm believes in him or herself. It is possible to change one's feeding habits, and it is possible to feel great about it. This is what you should convince yourself each day while on the program.

It is common to encounter people who discourage you whenever you are making life adjustments. These people will do everything possible to sabotage your endeavors so that you do not succeed. There are also those will entice you to go against you newly acquired habits and disciplines by telling you things such as that what you are doing is no way to live. Such individuals may make you feel horrible as if you weren't living to the fullest. It is thus important that you shun everything that they tell you and have firm believe in your new way of living. Do not permit anyone to persuade you that what you are doing is not right.

Wipe away negative thoughts

In addition to all these, you must set yourself free from negative thinking. Such thoughts as 'it's of no use, or this is only temporary should be buried in an unmarked grave deep in the forest of forgetfulness. Keep reminding yourself that you are new person following the new Beyond Diet Program and that negative thoughts do not have any place in you.

With the Beyond diet, it is advised that every negative thought that you have should be replaced with a positive thought. Thoughts of failures should be changed into thoughts of success, and any thoughts of doubt should be changed into thoughts of confidence.

Be Committed

It is not easy to commit to new lifestyle adjustments. However, the success of this program is pegged on undying devotion to see the program work. Besides the lifestyle changes that you ought to make, you will have to develop a strong commitment to achieve your weight goals and health objectives through the Beyond Diet program. This will require work, dedication, and unyielding commitment.

Goal Setting and Affirmations

The developer of the Beyond Diet program advises that for the program to work, there are three affirmations that ought to be chosen. The affirmations help you feel terrific about being in the program and encourage you to keep going. They are motivations to keep going on your new eating habits.

The three affirmations are:

1. I'm confident, disciplined and can achieve whatever I desire

2. Fresh, wholesome food, when consumed, will make me look and feel amazing

3. I love life, and each day of my life is a wonderful blessing

Of course, you do not have to go all nuts proclaiming these affirmations until people suspect that you have lost it. You merely have to repeat these affirmations quietly to yourself. Of course, the affirmations had better be backed by personal goals that you hope to achieve from the program.

It is advised that you write down these affirmations and carry them with you wherever you go. Anytime you are plagued with negative thoughts simply pull out the copy of your affirmations, and you will gradually feel the faith in the program gradually return. Most people who benefit from the program repeat their affirmations every morning and every evening.

Steps to Weight Loss

The Beyond Diet program is efficient in helping folks lose undesirable weight. However, it is one condition that requires that one is committed and puts in lots of hard work. The work to be done is however quite manageable and can broadly be grouped into three:

- First work out your metabolism

- Next create an ideal meal plan

- And finally learn the healthy foods to choose

The three steps are simple yet they will equip you with tools that lead to long-term weight loss and health benefits.

Working out your metabolism

We're all exceptional in our own unique designs including how our bodies function. This, therefore, translates into our bodies requiring different portions of proteins, fats and carbohydrates to work optimally. The way our body functions can be described as our unique metabolism type.

It is essential to learn your metabolism type since this helps you lose weight safely and in a healthy way. By adjusting to your metabolism type, you attain maximum wellness that last forever. This will be achieved without starvation and cravings that are present in most other diet plans.

Beginners who are trying to work out their metabolism plans must first understand this:

1. What's your type: carbohydrate, protein or mixed - depending on your body chemistry you can work out what are the ideal portions of healthy proteins, carbs, and fats that your body requires

2. The body's requirements for appropriate portions of healthy nutrients exist along a rather constant spectrum

3. Profiling of metabolism personalities is not a new phenomenon; doctors and nutritionists have been using it for decades to overcome lifestyle diseases such as obesity.

The success of a diet plan, in helping you lose weight and live better, is dependent on your metabolism type. This is why it is impractical to prescribe the same diet plan for different people with different metabolism types.

Similarly, certain foods are only ideal for certain metabolism types. Just because a particular food is healthy does not mean that it is healthy for people of all metabolism profiles.

This, therefore, implies that learning your metabolism profile is an essential facet to be considered when planning your meals. It helps you discover what foods are ideal for your metabolism and in what ratios they should be consumed. This is why most experts in weight loss begin their weight loss programs by first before all things typing the metabolism profile of the patient.

Chapter 2. Creating a Personal Meal Plan

After you have known your metabolism type you can now commence to work out how best to use the nutritional resources available to create a meal plan that will be effective in helping you achieve long-last weight loss and good health.

The Beyond Diet plan allows you to take into account your recommended calorie intake for your metabolism type and to track daily food intake and compare it to the effect it has on you. With time, one is able to determine the ideal foods for his or her metabolism and take them in the right portions. Therefore ideally you will be able to create your very own personalized Diet Solution Meal Plan.

Choosing the Best Foods

With a clearly determined metabolism type in place and a properly developed meal plan, one can now begin to identify the best foods to consume. Since the guideline in the Beyond Diet plan is completely natural it saves you time spent deciding whether the nutrients are healthy or not.

The natural foods that are included in the program will cut across all food groups and provide all the nutrients required for every metabolism profile in existence. The program incorporates fresh, unprocessed vegetables, fruits, nuts seeds, grains and unadulterated dairy, meat and fat products.

Artificial products range from packaged foods, cakes, cookies, frozen meals, artificial sweeteners, hydrogenated oils and high-fructose corn syrup among many others.

The Role of the Liver

It is imperative to watch what one eats. However to further qualify this statement it is important to consider the role of the liver.

As the body's largest organ, the liver is charged with carrying out processes that sustain life and promote health. It has an incredible role in weight loss and weight management since it is integral to innumerable metabolic process, control of blood sugar and digestive functions of the alimentary canal.

In managing weight, the liver is a critical organ since it has an important role in the biochemical breakdown of all that enters the body. It distinguishes between what nutrients to be assimilated into the body and what dangerous substances to be disintegrated and excreted. Sometimes whatever we eat is recognized as toxins. Such things as artificial sweeteners and other chemicals found in food are toxins that impair the liver's functions of processing nutrient and fats. This impairment is what leads to weight gain.

Bile a substance produced by the liver has various roles including breaking down fats and assimilating vitamins that are fat soluble. It also has another important role in detoxifying the body. In performing its detoxification duties, it may get clogged by toxins, and thus its functions get impaired. Such bile is thick viscous and inefficient in detoxifying the body.

Toxins additionally irritate the digestive system hence complications such as bloating and constipation. When stored in the body particularly in the fat cells, toxins impair various cell functions which may lead to cell death and destruction. They also create an acid milieu in the body which is ideal for growth of fungi, bacteria, viruses, parasites and other pathogens. A body that is linden with toxins loses its ability to metabolize fat and process it effectively leading to weight gain issues.

Chapter 3. Metabolism Types and Recommendations

Each person is unique. You must, therefore, understand your metabolism type better for the Beyond Diet plan to be effective for you. However, even after you have identified your metabolism type, you still might have to fine-tune your diet as you adjust your eating habits. Your body, however, will give you cues which you should pay attention to and with time you will understand exactly what your body needs. It is common for individuals to fall out of sync with their bodies such that they do not know how to it feels to be truly healthy.

Protein Type Metabolism

When you are a protein type metabolism person, you will typically crave foods that are rich and fatty. Such include foods like pizza, salty roasted nuts, and sausages. Most protein type metabolism people love food. Such people are rarely satisfied with a mere snack and will often feel famished even after large meals.

Eating carbohydrates gives such people sugar cravings. Once they begin eating sugary foods, they find it hard to stop. However, this makes them jittery and will make them hypoglycemic suddenly.

Most protein type metabolism people find it hard to lose weight through calorie-cutting methods. This often leads to misery since even with drastic decrease in calorie intake; their weight does not seem to improve.

A protein type will often notice energy problems when he or she eats the wrong food. Some feel extremely fatigued while others have that 'on edge' feeling. When such a person is nervous or anxious, they tend to eat since this makes them feel better. However, the relief does not last long as they will tend to feel worse soon afterward. They experience cycles of energy up and energy down often as a sign of mismatched food consumption and metabolism type.

What Protein Types Need

A protein type needs food rich in proteins and fat but low in carbs. Nonetheless, they still can eat carbohydrates in form of grains, vegetables, and fruits as long as they strike a balance with fats and proteins.

Protein types metabolize food faster than other metabolism types hence feel hungrier faster and more frequently. Their ideal meal planning should thus be inclusive of heavier protein choices that have high fat content. Such foods include whole eggs, dark meat, and dairy products. If protein types fail to eat such foods, they remain hungry all day and often struggle with their weight. They will also feel fatigued and anxious without cause.

Tips for Protein Types

Consume proteins- ensure that every meal or snack has protein especially animal protein.

Eat small but frequent meals- if a protein type does not eat often, low blood sugar will hit then hard. If it is not possible to eat frequently, then snacks that are rich in protein should be eaten in-between meals.

Stay away from refined carbs- foods that are rich in refined sugars such as bread and pastas can be incredibly disruptive for protein types.

Keep off most fruit juices and fruits- in spite of the promise of health that fruits hold, protein types have to be exceedingly cautious with their fruit selections. This is because most fruits are promptly converted into sugars which are rapidly absorbed into the bloodstream and well as we know sugar doesn't really go well with protein types. The finest fruit selections for protein types are apples and avocadoes

Carb types

Carb types have weak appetites. They can get by on amazingly small portions of food and will rarely think of food unless they are hungry. This is a class of most diagnosed workaholics. They are people who will not eat simply because they have no time for food. They are people who constantly send their metabolism on starvation mode for prolonged durations.

Their lifestyle often makes then prone to obesity and other weight management issues. Carb types are often dependent on caffeinated beverages that they bank on to keep them going. This dependency, unfortunately, may compound their already weakened appetite into an even worse nutritional condition.

Carb types have an unusually high tolerance for foods that are baked as well as vegetables that are starchy. This makes them over-eat these carbs which is a foundation for unhealthy conditions such as diabetes and obesity.

What Carb types need

More carbohydrates and less fats and proteins is what an ideal diet for a carb type personality should contain. The car types only require lighter low-fat proteins like white meat in their daily diets. They can, however, choose from a wide assortment of carbs and consume them in large quantities without any health or weight concerns.

Tips for carb types

Low-fat proteins are the best- eating high-fat proteins often leads to lethargy, fatigue and often depression

Consume dairy products cautiously- carb types have low tolerance for dairy products and tend to metabolize them poorly.

Be careful with your carb intake- low-starch vegetables should be consumed in plenty, and the ingestion of high-starch foods should be controlled. High-carbohydrate foods including bread and pasta tend to make you sleepy and sluggish.

Watch your legumes- it is not easy for carb types to easily digest all the proteins in legumes. It is thus recommended that they limit their legume intake.

Limit nuts and seeds since they add the fat content in a meal

Mixed Type Metabolism

These are people who require an equal proportion of protein, healthy fats, and carbohydrates. This makes it a very easy plan to manage since the food choices for these people are greater. Their appetite varies greatly; they may be ravenous at meals though not in between meals. Sometimes they may have a good appetite while on other occasions their appetite may be low. They rarely suffer craving however they tend to eat too much sugar.

For mixed types, the diet must incorporate high and low starch diets with high and low-fat proteins. Such a person must, therefore, familiarize him or herself with his or her body's requirements so as to know what works best for him or her

Calories

It is hard to discuss issues of weight loss without mentioning calories. It is important to understand that calorie is a unit of measurement of the energy released from food. Therefore, the body does need calories to perform its normal functions.

Low-calorie diets may bring about weight loss, but they also attract many other health problems such as breakdown of muscles and heart problems. This is because the diet fails to supply adequate energy to all the organs of the body.

Losing weight the healthy way, therefore, does not necessarily mean that one eats less. Though that may be a contributor to weight loss, losing weight should best be about adjusting your eating habits so that you offer the body just the precise amount of energy and prevent buildup of fat.

Daily Calorie Requirements

The Beyond diet program advises that one is able to work out his or her daily calorie requirements for improved benefits. One should know how many calories are enough to offer his or her body sufficient energy to perform all of its normal activities.

A good way of determining your daily calorie requirement is by multiplying your current weight in pounds by you level of activity(whether 13, 14 or 15 with 15 being vigorous activity and 13 being little or no exercise.) This gives you a healthy weight maintenance caloric intake. However, for weight loss, the maintenance calorie intake must be reduced by 20%.

Nevertheless, these calorie requirements are merely guidelines rather that hard-fixed rules that must be followed to the letter. Some individuals lose weight with fewer calories while others need more calories to lose weight healthily.

Daily Meal Planning

When one has already identified the ideal daily calorie intake as well as their metabolism type, it is now easy to plan your daily diet.

Ideal Protein-Carb-Fat Ratios

A carb type person should consume on average 70% carbs, 20% protein and 10% fats while protein type people should eat approximately 45% protein, 20% fats, and 35% carbohydrates. Mixed type people have a wider margin for their eating requirements, but the recommended intake should be about 50% carbohydrates, 40% proteins, and 10% fats. An easier means of looking at it is that for a mixed type metabolism, each meal or snack should be approximately half protein and half carbohydrates.

The Ideal Food Servings

This should be guided by your recommended daily calorie intake and your metabolism type. There is a menu that is available for members at the Beyond Diet official website that helps one determine the ideal servings for each meal.

Identifying the Ideal Meals

Eating the proper type of food is just as important as it eating the right portions of food daily. A chart is also available on the official website of Beyond Diet Plan to help in   easy identification of the best food choices for various metabolism types. Personal preferences too should be considered since one ought to feel good about the food that he or she is eating.

Planning Your Meals

Once you have put together all the necessary information, you can now begin drawing up your personalized meal plan. For instance, if you are a protein person, your breakfast should have a single carbohydrate service which could be a cup of cooked oatmeal or a medium sized apple. Your ideal snack should have one carbohydrate and three protein servings; you can thus have 1½ounce raw almonds and a medium sized apple or 3oz leftover turkey and ½ cup each of carrots and celery.

Following the guide on ideal servings and ideal foods plan a worksheet for each day's meals and snacks. For snacks, it is essential to avoid some of the unhealthy, empty calorie snacks that are commonly available such as candy and chips. Healthier alternatives such as nuts and raw fruits should be chosen.

Your plan for meals should be inclusive of fats. Many folks who are struggling to shed unwanted weight tend to overlook fats believing that fats impede healthy loss of weight. Not all fat is bad. Healthy fats, when consumed in the right quantities, will help you feel satiated, with high energy levels and eventually help you lose weight.

Chapter 4. Recipes

Here are some delicious recipe options for your Beyond Diet Plan. There are other numerous recipes for tasty, healthy and easy to prepare meals that can be found online. We also urge you to be creative in your cooking as long as you stay healthy in what you eat.

Rainbow Quinoa for Breakfast

This is a tasty breakfast option that makes you supercharged for the day

What You Need:

0.25c black organic quinoa

0.75c white organic quinoa

1fresh organic garlic cloves

1fresh medium-sized red organic tomato

1 fresh organic celery stalk

0.25c fresh organic carrot

0.25c fresh organic bell pepper (green, red and yellow)

1fresh organic green onion

2 omega-3 cage-free organic whole eggs

½ tablespoon unrefined pure sea salt.

1 tablespoon unrefined, unfiltered, extra virgin olive oil

Method

The vegetables and quinoa are combined with 2 cups of water in a saucepan.

Salt, garlic, and the olive oil are added, and the mixture brought to boil.

The heat is lowered, and the saucepan covered. The combination is let to simmer for about 10 minutes until the water evaporates.

2 tablespoons of olive oil are heated in a frying pan.

The eggs added into the pan and cooked, scrabbling till they are done.

The cooked quinoa is added into the pan and stirred in.

The mixture is covered and cooked for about 10 minutes.

When ready, it is served with sliced tomato.

Basic Roasted Chicken for Dinner

The recipe is quick and easy. The chicken is delicious and leftovers can be frozen or refrigerated for quick meals within the week

What You Need:

2 tablespoons fresh organic thyme

1 fresh organic garlic cloves

1 tablespoon raw unsalted grass-fed, organic butter

¾ teaspoon pure unrefined sea salt

½ organic black pepper ground

6lbs raw whole chicken skinned

Method

The oven is preheated to 350°F.

The chicken is washed and fat removed from inside cavities.

The softened butter, salt, pepper, minced garlic, and thyme are combined in a small bowl into a paste.

The paste is rubbed onto the chicken.

The chicken is put into a roasting pan breast side down; roast the chicken uncovered basting frequently for about 90 minutes.

The chicken is ready when it is pricked with a fork and no juices run red and when the legs pull off easily.

Take the chicken from the pan and let it rest for 5-10 minutes while covered.

Cut the chicken into serving pieces.

The roasting pan may be deglazed to make gravy which if desired can be thickened with 1½ Tbsp. of arrowroot powder mixed with 2 cups of water.

Shrimps and Spicy Peanut Sauce for Lunch

What You Need

1fresh organic basil

1large organic red onion

1fresh organic orange

6 fresh organism garlic cloves

2 tablespoons fresh organic ginger

2 cups organic brown rice

12 cooked wild-caught shrimps

2 tablespoons unrefined, unfiltered extra virgin organic olive oil

2 tablespoons raw, unfiltered organic honey

4 tablespoons creamy raw organic peanut butter

½ teaspoon organic chili powder

Pure unrefined sea salt

½ teaspoon organic cayenne pepper powder

Method

The rice is put in a pot with water and boiled.

The onion is chopped into tiny pieces.

About 2 tablespoons of olive oil are heated up in a saucepan of medium size and 2/3 of the chopped onion added.

5 cloves of the garlic are chopped and added into the pan and sautéed till the onion starts to brown.

The peeled, frozen shrimps are added into the pan and sautéed till they are done.

The remaining onion is put into a blender; the ginger, reaming garlic cloves and about 3 tablespoons of water are also added in. the blender is turned on for a few seconds. The peanut butter, honey, chili powder, cayenne pepper and about 4 leaves of basil are added to the blender. The juice of ½ orange is also added, and the blender turned on again for a few seconds.

The spicy peanut sauce is mixed with the shrimps in the saucepan and seasoned with salt.

The meal is ready to serve and can be garnished with fresh basil and orange.

Conclusion

The Beyond Diet plan offers an ideal way of optimizing health without starvation and cravings. It is more of a toolkit towards optimum health and ideal weight while still enjoying food. It is easy to modify the plan, and you will definitely feel good when on the program.

Thank You Page

I want to personally thank you for reading my book. I hope you found information in this book useful and I would be very grateful if you could leave your honest review about this book. I certainly want to thank you in advance for doing this.

If you have the time, you can check my other books too.

Lightning Source UK Ltd.
Milton Keynes UK
UKOW06f1838250815

257528UK00016B/438/P